100% NATURAL WAYS TO TREAT LEUKEMIA

Leukemia (Deadly Disease)

Dr.BAYO

TABLE OF CONTENTS

Introduction

Leukemia is referring to as the cancer of the blood or bone marrow.   Bone marrow manufactures blood cells. Leukemia can occur when there is an issue with the manufacturing of blood cells. It is normallty affects the leukocytes, or white blood cells.

It is most common to the people over the age of 55 years, but it is also the most common cancer in those aged less than 15 years.

In the United States, 62,130 people are beleived to receive a diagnosis of leukemia in 2017, and around 24,500 deaths will likely be because of this disease.

Acute leukemia grows quickly and worsens speedly, but chronic leukemia gets deadly over time.

The outlook for people with leukemia can be decided on the type.

Every patient who is going through remission will need to go through a regular check up, added blood tests and possible bone marrow tests, to be sure the cancer has not returned.

If the leukemia does not comes back, the physician may decide, over time, to decrease the frequency of the tests.

Leukemia is normally thought of as a children's condition, but it actually seeing in adults. It's more rampant in men than women and more in whites than African-Americans.

There's really nothing you can do to prevent leukemia. It's cancer of your blood cells caused by a high in the number of white blood cells in your body. They crowd out the red blood cells and platelets your body needs to be healthy. All those extra white blood cells don't work right, and that causes problems.

Chapter One

WHAT IS LEUKEMIA?

Leukemia is a malignancy (cancer) of blood cells.

In leukemia, abnormal blood cells are produced in the
bone marrow. Normally, leukemia affects the production
of abnormal white blood cells, the cells responsible for
combating infection. However, the abnormal cells in
leukemia is not active in the same way as normal white
blood cells. The leukemia cells continue to increase and
split, eventually crowding out the original blood cells.
The end result is that it becomes difficult for the body to
combat infections, control bleeding, and transport
oxygen.

History of Leukemia

Leukemia, a malignant cancer of the blood, was called in
1847 by Dr. Rudolf Virchow, a German politician whose
broad-ranging interests led him to significant researches
in cell biology, pathology and anthropology. Although
Dr. Virchow's name showned often in The New York
Times, mostly in the late 19th century, his foundings
about leukemia was not mentioned until Feb. 22, 1970,
in an article by Dr. Lawrence K. Altman.

However, that was not the first time the ailment was mentioned in the paper. That occur on Dec. 6, 1899, when Maj. Samuel T. Armstrong, surgeon of the 32nd Infantry, died in Manila. "The cause of death," the brief obituary said, "is given as leukemia."

By 1913, various types of leukemia were revealed, although none were curable. On Dec. 2 of that year, The Times mentioned the ailment in a report on the death of a Cornell student "suffering from a grave blood disease described by the hospital authorities as chronic lymphatic leukemia." This was also the first mention of an attempt to cure the ailment with a blood transfusion from the patient's twin brother.

The next failed cured noted in the paper was radium. On May 3, 1915, The Times reported that radium "has also been found active in leukemia," but then acknowledged that.
"Patients might even succumb to the poisons released into the system." Still, this was the first mention of a treatment, radiation therapy that today remains one of the treatments for the illness.

Different types of leukemia

Leukemias are further grouped as myeloid or lymphoid, depending upon the type of white blood cell that makes up the leukemia cells. A basic understanding of the normal growth of blood cells is needed to understand the numerous types of leukemia. Main blood cells grow from stem cells that have the potential to become vast cell types. Myeloid stem cells develop in the bone marrow and become immature white cells called myeloid blasts. These myeloid blasts further mature to become either red blood cells, platelets, or certain kinds of white blood cells. Lymphoid stem cells mature in the bone marrow to become lymphoid blasts. The lymphoid blasts develop further into T or B lymphocytes (T-cells or B-cells), special types of white blood cells. Myeloid or myelogenous leukemias are made up of cells that arise from myeloid cells, while lymphoid leukemias arise from lymphoid cells. Knowing the type of cell involved in leukemia is vital in choosing the appropriate cure.

Common types of leukemia

The four most common types of leukemia are acute lymphocytic leukemia, chronic lymphocytic leukemia, acute myeloid leukemia, and chronic myeloid leukemia.

- Acute lymphocytic leukemia (ALL, also refer to as acute lymphoblastic leukemia) is the most significant type of leukemia in Adolescent, but it can also affect adults. In this type of leukemia, immature lymphoid cells increase speedly in the blood. It affects almost 6,000 people per year in the U.S.
- Acute myeloid leukemia (AML, also refered to as acute myelogenous leukemia) this has to do with the speedy development of myeloid cells. It happens in both adults and children and affects about 19,500 people each year in the U.S.
- Chronic lymphocytic leukemia (CLL) this is a slow developing cancer of lymphoid cells that usually affects people over 55 years of age. It is estimated to have impacts in about 21,000 people in the U.S. every year. It almost never happens in children or adolescents.
- Chronic myeloid leukemia (CML, also known as chronic myelogenous leukemia) is a type of chronic myeloproliferative disorder that primarily affects adults and happens in about 8,400 people every year in the U.S.

Lower common types of leukemia account for about 6,000 cases of leukemia each year in the U.S.

- Hairy cell leukemia is an uncommon type of chronic leukemia.
- Chronic myelomonocytic leukemia (CMML) is another type of chronic leukemia that grows from myeloid cells.
- Juvenile myelomonocytic leukemia (JMML) is a type of myeloid leukemia that usually happens in adolescent less than 6 years of age.
- Wide granular lymphocytic leukemia (LGL leukemia) is a type of chronic leukemia that grows from lymphoid cells. It can be slow- or fast-developing.

Acute promyelocytic leukemia (APL) is a subtype of AML

Chapter Two

Fast fact on leukemia

Exposure to radiation is known to high the risk of growing AML, CML, or ALL. High rates of leukemia were observed in people surviving atomic bombs. Radiation therapy for cancer cans also high the risk of leukemia. Getting involved with some chemicals, comprising benzene (used commonly in the chemical industry), high the risk of leukemia. Smoking of cigarrette is known to high the risk of developing AML.

Some genetic disorders can high the risk; Down syndrome, Li-Fraumeni syndrome, and some other medical conditions can high the risk of growing leukemia. Blood disorders known as myelodysplastic syndromes confer can high the risk of growing AML. Human T-cell leukemia virus type 1 (HTLV-1) is a virus that causes a rare type of leukemia.

Some chemotherapy drugs for cancer can high the risk for AML or ALL.

Having risk factors does not determine that a person wills definitely contacted leukemia, and many people with risk factors will not grow the ailment. Likewise, not everyone who grows leukemia has an identifiable risk factor.

Symptoms and signs of leukemia

The symptoms and signs of leukemia is determined upon the type of leukemia. As stated earlier, slow-developing or chronic leukemia may not cause any symptoms at the outset, while aggressive or speedily developing leukemia may lead to chronic symptoms. The signs of leukemia arise from a loss of function of the normal blood cells or from accumulation of the abnormal cells in the body.

Signs and symptoms of leukemia typically consist of the following:

- Fevers
- Night sweats
- Swollen lymph nodes that are usually painless
- Feelings of fatigue, tiredness

- Easy bleeding or bruising, causing bluish or purplish patches on the skin or tiny red spots on the skin, or recurring nosebleeds
- Frequent infections
- Bone or joint pain
- Weight loss that is unintentional and otherwise unexplained, or loss of appetite
- Enlargement of the spleen or liver, which can lead to abdominal pain or swelling
- Red spots on the skin (petechiae)

If leukemia cells have infiltrated the brain, symptoms such as headaches, seizures, confusion, loss of muscle control, and vomiting can happen.

Causes of leukemia

The main cause of leukemia is not known, but it is thought to indulge a combination of genetic and environmental factors. Leukemia cells have acquired mutations in their DNA that cause them to develop abnormally and lose functions of typical white blood cells. It is not clear what causes these mutations to happen. One aspect of change in the cells' DNA that is popular in leukemias is known as a chromosome translocation. In this process, a portion of one chromosome breaks off and joined to a various chromosome. One translocation seen in almost all cases of CML and in sometimes in other types of leukemia is an exchange of DNA between chromosomes 9 and 22, which results to what is known as the Philadelphia chromosome. This creates an oncogene (cancer-promoting gene) known as BCR-ABL. This transformed in DNA is not inherited but happens sometime in the life of the affected personality.

Most cases of leukemia are not believed to be hereditary, but some genetic mutations and conditions can be given along to offspring that high the chances of growing leukemia. A condition known as Li-Fraumeni syndrome is characterized by an inherited mutation in a tumor suppressor gene known as TP53, and individuals with this condition have a high risk of leukemia and other cancers. Other hereditary conditions that can high the risk of growing leukemia consist of: Down syndrome, neurofibromatosis

type 1, ataxia telangiectasia, and Noonan syndrome.

Chapter Three

How does medical personnel diagnonise leukemia?

Hematologists are specialist medical personnel who diagnose and cure blood diseases, comprising leukemia; hematologist-oncologists cure blood diseases like leukemia, as well as other diffrent cancers.

In addition to a medical history, asking about symptoms and risk factors and a physical exam to search for signs of leukemia (lymph node enlargement, enlargement of spleen), the diagnosis of leukemia typically has to do with the laboratory discovery of a blood sample. Abnormal numbers of blood cells may determine a diagnosis of leukemia, and the blood sample may also be investigated under the microscope to see if the cells show abnormal. A sample of the bone marrow may also be derived to start the diagnosis. For a bone marrow aspirate, a long, thin needle is used to remove a sample of bone marrow from the hip bone, under local anesthesia. A bone marrow biopsy has to do with insertion of a thick, hollow needle into the hip bone to withdraw a sample of the bone marrow, using local anesthesia.

Cells from the blood and bone marrow are further examined if leukemia cells are present. This additional examination search for genetic alterations and expression of some cell surface markers by the cancer cells (immunophenotyping). The results of these exams are used to aid to decide the exact classification of the leukemia and to determined on optimal cured.

Other exams that may be needful comprise of a chest X-ray to decide if there are enlarged lymph nodes or other signs of disease and a lumbar puncture to withdraw a sample of cerebrospinal fluid to decide if the leukemia cells have infiltrated the membranes and space surrounding the brain and spinal cord.

However, exams such as MRI and CT scanning can also be needful for some patients to decide the extent of disease.

What are treatment options for leukemia?

There are a number of various medical approaches to the treatment or cure for leukemia. Cure will be typically determine upon the type of leukemia, the patient's age and health condition, as well as whether or not the leukemia cells have spread to the cerebrospinal fluid. The genetic changes or specific features of the leukemia cells as decided in the laboratory can also decided the type of medication that may be most suitable.

Carefully waiting may be an option for a lot of people with a chronic leukemia who do not have symptoms. This has to do with close attentively of the disease so that the cure can start when symptoms grows. Carefully waiting release the patient to avoid or shift the side impacts of treatment. The risk of carefullness is that it may removed the possibility of controlling the leukemia before it worsens.

Cures for leukemia include chemotherapy, major treatment modality for leukemia, radiation therapy, biological therapy, targeted therapy, and stem cell transplant. Additional of these treatments may be used. Surgical elimination of the spleen can be a part of treatment if the spleen is widened.

Acute leukemia needs to be cured when it is diagnosed, with the aim of inducing a remission (absence of leukemia cells in the body). After remission is achieved, therapy may be applied to stop a relapse of the leukemia. This is called consolidation or maintenance therapy. Acute leukemias can often be cured with treatment.

Chronic leukemias are unlikely to be cured with treatment, but treatments are often able to control the cancer and manage symptoms. Some people with chronic leukemia may be candidates for stem cell transplantation, which does offer a chance for cure.

Many patients opt to get a second thought before starting treatment for leukemia. In most cases, there is time to receive a second thought and choosed a treatment options without making the treatment less active. In addition, rare cases of very aggressive leukemias, treatment must start immediately. One should have a talk with medical personnel on the possibility of getting a second thought and any potential delays in treatment. Most physicians entertained the possibility of a second thought and should not be offended by a patient's wish to get one.

1. Chemotherapy

Chemotherapy is the administration of drugs that kill rapidly dividing cells such as leukemia or other cancer cells. Chemotherapy may be taken orally in pill or tablet form, or it may be delivered via a catheter or intravenous line directly into the bloodstream. Combination chemotherapy is usually given, which involves a combination of more than one drug. The drugs are given in cycles with rest periods in between.

Sometimes, chemotherapy drugs for leukemia are delivered directly to the cerebrospinal fluid (known as intrathecal chemotherapy). Intrathecal chemotherapy is given in addition to other types of chemotherapy and can be used to cure leukemia in the brain or spinal cord or, in some cases, to stop the spread of leukemia to the brain and spinal cord. An Ommaya reservoir is a special catheter put under the scalp for the delivery of chemotherapy medications. This is used for adolescent and some adult patients as a way to rejects injections into the cerebrospinal fluid.

Side effects of chemotherapy determined on the particular drugs taken and the dosage or regimen. Some side effects from chemotherapy drugs comprises of hair loss, nausea, vomiting, mouth sores, loss of appetite, tiredness, easy bruising or bleeding, and a high chance of infection because of the destruction of white blood cells. There are medications obtainable to help manage the side effects of chemotherapy.

Some adult men and women who receive chemotherapy sustain damage to the ovaries or testes, resulting in infertility. Most adolescent who receive chemotherapy for leukemia will have normal fertility as adults, but depending on the drugs and dosages used, some may have infertility as adults.

2. Biological therapy

Biological therapy is any treatment that uses living organisms, substances that come from living organisms, or synthetic versions of these substances to treat cancer. These treatments help the immune system recognize abnormal cells and then attack them. Biological therapies for numerous types of cancer can comprise of antibodies, tumor vaccines, or cytokines (substances that are produced within the body to control the immune system). Monoclonal antibodies are antibodies that react against a specific target that are used in the treatment of different kinds of cancer. An example of a monoclonal antibody used in the treatment of leukemia is alemtuzumab, which targets the CD52 antigen, a protein found on B-cell chronic lymphocytic leukemia (CLL) cells. Interferons are cell signaling chemicals that have been used in the treatment of leukemia.

Side effects of biological therapies tend to be low chronic than those of chemotherapy and can include rash or swelling at the injection site for IV infusions of the therapeutic agents. Other side effects can include headache, muscle aches, **fever**, or tiredness.

3. Targeted therapy

Targeted therapies are drugs that interfere with one specific property or function of a cancer cell, rather than acting to kill all speedily developing cells indiscriminately. This means there is low damage to normal cells with targeted therapy than with chemotherapy. Targeted therapies may cause the target cell to cease developing rather than to die, and they interfere with specific molecules that promote development or spread of cancers. Targeted cancer therapies are also referred to as molecularly targeted drugs, molecularly targeted therapies, or precision medicines.

Monoclonal antibodies (described above in the section on biologic therapy) are also considered to be targeted therapies since they specifically interfere and interact with a specific target protein on the surface of cancer cells. Imatinib (Gleevec) and dasatinib (Sprycel) are examples of targeted therapies that are used to cure CML, some cases of ALL, and some other cancers. These drugs target the cancer-promoting protein that is formed by the BCR-ABL gene translocation.

Targeted therapies are given in pill form or by injection. Side effects can include swelling, bloating, and sudden weight gain. Other side effects can include nausea, vomiting, diarrhea, muscle cramps, or rash.

4. Radiation therapy

Radiation therapy uses high energy radiation to target cancer cells. Radiation therapy may be used in the treatment of leukemia that has spread to the brain, or it may be used to target the spleen or other areas where leukemia cells have accumulated.

Radiation therapy also causes side effects, but they are not likely to be permanent. Side effects depend on the location of the body that is irradiated. For example, radiation to the abdomen can cause nausea, vomiting, and diarrhea. With any radiation therapy, the skin in the area being treated may become red, dry, and tender. Generalized tiredness is also common while undergoing radiation therapy.

5. Stem cell transplant

In stem cell transplantation, high doses of chemotherapy and/or radiation are given to destroy leukemia cells along with normal bone marrow. Then, transplant stem cells are delivered by an intravenous infusion. The stem cells travel to the bone marrow and start producing new blood cells. Stem cells may come from the patient or from a donor.

Autologous stem cell transplantation is known to be a situation in which the patient's own stem cells are removed and treated to spoil leukemia cells. They are then returned to the body after the bone marrow and leukemia cells have been destroyed.

An allogeneic stem cells transplant refers to stem cells transplanted from a donor. These may be from a relative or an unrelated donor. A syngeneic stem cell transplant uses stem cells taken from a healthy identical twin of the patient.

Stem cells may be removed (harvested) in various ways. Typically, they are taken from the blood. They can also be harvested from the bone marrow or from umbilical cord blood.

Stem cell transplantation is done in a hospital, and it is necessary to stay in the hospital for several weeks. Risks of the procedure comprises of infections and bleeding because of the depletion of normal blood cells. A risk of stem cell transplant with donor cells is known as graft-versus-host disease (GVHD). In GVHD, the donor white blood cells react against the patient's normal tissues. GVHD can be mild or very severe, and often affects the liver, skin, or digestive tract. GVHD can happen at any time after the transplant, even years later. Steroids or medications that limit the immune response may be used to treat this complication.

6. Chimeric antigen receptor (CAR) T-cell treatment

Chimeric antigen receptor (CAR) T-cell treatment is a new form of treatment in which a patient's own normal T lymphocytes are re-engineered in a laboratory to attack the leukemia cells and are then reintroduced into the patient's bloodstream. This treatment has been used for people with B-cell **lymphomas** that have relapsed or are refractory to treatment. It is also an endorsed treatment option for some cases of leukemia. The U.S. FDA approved tisagenlecleucel (Kymriah) in 2018 for the treatment of patients up to 25 years of age with B-cell precursor acute lymphoblastic leukemia (ALL) that is refractory or in second or later relapse.

CAR-T therapy is also available in clinical trials. Cytokine-release syndrome (CRS) is a potentially serious side effect frequently associated with CAR T-cell therapy. Cytokines are chemical messengers produced when the CAR T-cells multiply in the body and kill cancer cells. CRS may cause a range of symptoms from mild flu-like symptoms to more serious symptoms including fast heart rate, low blood pressure, and heart problems. Other side effects can include nerve damage, suppressed immune function, and a condition known as tumor lysis syndrome that results when cancer cells are speedily destroyed.

Because CAR T-cell therapy is so new, the patients who have had this treatment have not been followed over the long term. Researches are under way to decide whether CAR-T treatment may be useful in other types of leukemia.

7. Supportive treatments

Due to numerous treatments for leukemia deplete normal blood cells, increasing the risk for bleeding and infection, supportive treatments may be needed to assist to stop these complications of treatment. Supportive treatments may also be needed to aid reduce and manage unpleasant side effects of medical or radiation therapy.

Types of supportive and preventive treatments that can be used for patients undergoing treatment for leukemia include the following:

- Vaccines against the flu or pneumonia
- Blood or platelet transfusions
- Anti-nausea medications
- Antibiotics or antiviral medications to treat or prevent infections
- White blood cell growth factors to stimulate white blood cell production (such as granulocyte-colony stimulating factor [G-CSF], made up of filgrastim [Neupogen] and pegfilgrastim [Neulasta] and granulocyte macrophage-colony stimulating growth factor [GM-CSF], comprises of of sargramostim[Leukine])
- Red cell growth factors to stimulate red blood cell production (darbepoetin alfa [Aranesp] or epoetin alfa [Procrit])
- Intravenous injections of immunoglobulins to help fight infection

Chapter Four

Complications of leukemia

Most of the challenges of leukemia relate to the depletion of normal blood cells as well as the side effects of treatments as described in the previous section, such as frequent infections, bleeding, and GVHD in recipients of stem cell transplants. Weight loss and anemia are further complications of leukemia and its treatment. Complications of any leukemia also comprise of a relapse or a progression of the disease after a remission has been achieved with treatment.

Other complications of leukemia relate to the specific type of leukemia. For example, in 3% to 5% of cases of CLL, the cells change characteristics and transform into an aggressive lymphoma. This is known as a Richter transformation. Autoimmune hemolytic anemic, in the body attacks and destroys red blood cells, is another potential complication of CLL. People with CLL are also more likely to grow second cancers and other blood disorders and blood cancers.

Tumor lysis syndrome is a condition caused by the quick death of cancer cells during acute treatment. It can happen in almost any type of cancer, and it is seen with some certain cases of leukemia, particularly when large numbers of leukemia cells are present such as with AML or ALL. The quick destruction of the leukemia cells leads to the release of large amounts of phosphate, which further causes metabolic abnormalities and can lead to kidney failure.

Children who receive therapy for ALL may experience late adverse effects including central nervous system (CNS) impairment, reducing the development, infertility, cataracts, and an increased risk for other cancers. The incidence of these late effects varies depending upon the age at treatment and the type and strength of therapies.

Prognosis of leukemia

The prognosis of leukemia is determined upon the type of leukemia that is present and the age and health status of the patient. Mortality (death) rates for leukemia are increased in the elderly than in younger adults and children. In many cases, leukemia can be managed or cured with treatments obtainable today. In particular, childhood ALL has a very high 5-year survival rate.

Modern treatments have led to a greater than fourfold increase since 1960 in five-year survival rates for leukemia. Five-year survival rates for different types of leukemia from 2007-2013 are approximately:

CML: 68%

CLL: 86%

AML: 27% overall, 66% for children and **teens** younger than 15

ALL: 71% overall, over 90% for children

About the *Author*

Dr. Bayo is a pastor and a medical practioner who studied pharmacy in SefakoMakgatho Health Sciences University (SMU) in South Africa and receive his Phd in Lipscomb University in Missouri-columbia.
He has involved himself into prescriptions and cure of diseases and sickness. He is a solution to many problems amidst its environment such has cancer, stroke infection, erectile dysfuntion, anti-biotic infection, how to reduce your blood pressure and lots more to mention but a little. He has been eagerly and greatly having impact in the life of msny others in the area of pharmaceutical trainings and has been building people to be pharmaceutically awake in order not to be deceived by fake drug sellers out there.

Acknowledgments

My appreciation goes to God, Almighty for the opportunity to collate this manuscript, and for wisdom he gave me to spread the knowledge around. Also I appreciate everyone that supported me during the compilation, proof reading and publishing of the book

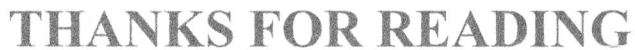

THANKS FOR READING

www.ingramcontent.com/pod-product-compliance
Lightning Source LLC
Chambersburg PA
CBHW071124220526

45467CB00004B/2044